I0101524

Your Amazing Itty Bitty® Health and Wellness Experts Compilation Book

15 Health & Wellness Professionals Share Essential Information on Areas of Their Expertise

Donna Bach & Gary Groesbeck
Sharon Barnard
Pat Buchanan
Deborah Chelette-Wilson
Karen Daniels
Debra Graugnard
Patty Hedrick

Zadra Ibañez
Joyce Khoury
Yvonne L Larson
Joanne Neweduk
Denise Schickel
Patricia Tanner
Denise Thomson
Ronni Zorn

Published by Itty Bitty® Publishing
A subsidiary of S & P Productions, Inc.

Printed in the United States of America

Itty Bitty Publishing
311 Main Street, Suite D
El Segundo, CA 90245
(310) 640-8885

ISBN: 978-1-950326-71-6

Health and Wellness Comes in Many Forms

15 Health & Wellness Professionals Share Essential Information on Areas of Their Expertise

In this Amazing Itty Bitty® Book fifteen experts combine to provide you with information about:

- Donna Bach & Gary Groesbeck - The Power of Neuro Alchemy; Flow to Awaken and Evolve Your Mind and Life
- Sharon Barnard - Change Your Breathing Change Your Life – 3 Minutes to Peace
- Pat Buchanan - Back Pain or Comfort – It's Your Choice
- Deborah Chelette-Wilson - Transforming Trauma Into Triumph
- Karen Daniels - Navigate Life With Inner Wisdom
- Debra Graugnard - Food, Weight & Famine Power
- Patty Hedrick - Your Roadmap to Active Aging
- Zadra Ibañez - All Essential Oils Are Not Created Equal
- Joyce Khoury - Understanding The Complicated Medicare Maze
- Yvonne L Larson - Mastering Your Zone
- Joanne Neweduk - Improving Your Life With Light
- Denise Schickel - Your Body
- Patricia Tanner - Young Living Essential Oils
- Denise Thomson - How Does Stress Increase Disease
- Ronni Zorn - Vital, Vibrant & Vivacious With Veggies

If you are interested in learning more about improving your health and overall wellness pick up a copy of this informative Itty Bitty® book today.

Dedications:

Donna Bach & Gary Groesbeck: Dedicated to the memory of our beloved mentor in "Awakened Mind" Coaching, Anna Wise, we are grateful to carry your torch.

Sharon Barnard: Beloved friend, I pray that you are prospering in every way and that you continually enjoy good health, just as your soul is prospering. 3 John 1:2 (The Passion Translation)

Pat Buchanan: To all my teachers. To all my relations. Deep bows to Moshe, Esther, and Thay.

Deborah Chelette-Wilson: To all my clients from ages 2 to 104 who taught me trauma knows no age limits and the human spirit is always open for healing.

Karen Daniels: With delight and love, I dedicate my inner wisdom chapter to my family, especially Dave, Byron, Kevin, and Maite, who share my belief in a life-long commitment to health and wellness.

Debra Graugnard: To the woman who longs to live fully embodied, safe in her skin, with empowerment, mastery, and freedom to BE true to her Sacred Self.

Patty Hedrick: This is for my mentors, family, and fellow entrepreneurs, who showed me that opportunities in nursing are endless and ever-changing.

Zadra Ibañez: Dedicated to Blujay and Amber, for all their guidance along the way.

Joyce Khoury: Thank you to my entire family for the unconditional support I receive from them in helping me to achieve my dreams. And…thank you to the universe for showing me there is always going to be a way to help our fellow human beings no matter what the issue is.

Yvonne L Larson: I dedicate this to Karen, Percy, and my three fur babies Miss Molly Waddles, Percy, and Fiona who each epitomized resilience. Thank you for your relentless, unconditional love.

Joanne Neweduk: To my beautiful blended family. Our love and laughter fills my soul.

Denise Schickel: This is chapter is dedicated to my clients.

Denise Thomson: I want to thank Suzy and Joan for guiding and encouraging me in the process of writing this chapter. Also thanks to my husband and daughter for pointing out my strengths, skills, and talents and for believing in me.

Patricia Tanner: To my friend Patricia Busch a fellow Reflexologist whose constant support in, and with the use of Essential Oils has been a blessing. She has been a true friend and supporter of all my efforts.

Ronni Zorn: To my mom, thanks for the gift of my Plant-Based Nutrition Certification program. Thank you to Drs. Campbell, Esselstyn, Barnard & Fuhrman, Luanne Pennessi, Gary Null, Robin Helfritch & her husband Demo; all of you have made a difference in my life.

Stop by our Itty Bitty® website Directory to find interesting Health and Wellness information from our experts.

www.IttyBittyPublishing.com

Or visit our Experts at:

Donna Bach and Gary Groesbeck
www.neuroalchemyflow.com

Sharon Barnard
Inhaleloveyoga.com
sharon@inhaleloveyoga.com

Pat Buchanan
www.DrPatBuchanan.com

Deborah Chelette-Wilson
deborahchelettewilson@gmail.com,
www.alifeofloveandbalance.com

Karen Daniels
www.windsongexpressivearts.com

Debra Graugnard
http://JoyfullyLiving.com

Patty Hedrick
www.mlhcc.com

Zadra Ibañez
http://greenucopia.com

Joyce Khoury
www.insurancecoachforyou.com

Yvonne L Larson
YvonneLynnLarson.com

Joanne Neweduk
www.FabulousHealth.ca

Denise Schickel
www.amazon.com/dp/1950326322

Patricia Tanner
MYYL.com/Tannerhealth

Denise Thomson
Coachdenise@ctdigest.net

Ronni Zorn
emergetothrive.com

Table of Contents

Expert 1
Donna Bach and Gary Groesbeck
The Power of Neuro Alchemy Flow to Awaken and Evolve Your Mind and Life

When life becomes difficult and you need relief from uncertainty and stress, Neuro Alchemy Flow coaching can be the most effective system to help you jump into effortless Flow states on demand.

1. You will learn to achieve the ideal ratios of brainwave patterns similar to dreaming, but while wide awake and operating efficiently.
2. Sourced from over 4 decades of research and practice, uniting the power of modern EEG neurofeedback, heart rhythm biofeedback technology, and the wisdom of ancient traditions, it brings about transformation of consciousness and awakening.
3. Practical directions and navigational tools assist you in accessing ease, comfort, and joy throughout the chaotic challenges of life. Private, groups or virtual trainings use the latest electronic brainwave (EEG) monitoring equipment called the "Mind Mirror." These states are "Brain hacks" to Flow.

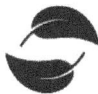

Benefits of Neuro Alchemy Training

- Discover the meaning of the five frequencies of brainwaves and how to produce them:
  (Gamma, Beta, Alpha, Theta, and Delta)
- Increase your brain's focus, productivity, and creativity by 300% while in Flow.
- Learn methods of "owning your own body" to increase the health of your heart, immune system, and moods.
- Adopt new strategies to experience bliss and euphoria combining secrets of ancient traditions and modern science, demystifying the mystical.
- The exercises you will practice invite you to deeply relax and discover the unlimited aspects of your authentic, deeper self.
- The entire step-by-step training with the virtual online course is accessible for remote training.

Expert 2
Sharon Barnard
Change Your Breathing, Change Your Life - 3 minutes to peace

Do you spend too much time at your desk: feeling stressed, tense & scattered? Staying confined in one place for so long can slow your energy down and keep yourself from being as productive as you can be.

1. Dr. James Levine, a professor of medicine at the Mayo Clinic calls "sitting; the new smoking" with health risks like increased chance of obesity, cardiovascular disease, increased rate of Type 2 diabetes, and loss of energy.
2. Being hunched in an office chair restricts your lung capacity and breathing.
3. Shallow breathing can lead to stress, stress can lead to anxiety.
4. Using just your mind all day can cause feelings of discontentment & anxiety.
5. Anxiety disorders are the most common mental illness in the US affecting 40 million adults.
6. You may be saying, "yes, yes, yes, but where do I start?"

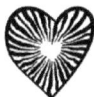

Just Breath

Allow your spine to belong and neutral from the tailbone to the crown of your head whether standing, sitting, or lying down. When you are in a stressed & anxious state, breathing becomes shallow. As you intentionally slow your breath down & inflate your lungs fully, you will:

- Connect mind & body bringing peace
- Switch from "fight or flight" mode to "rest & digest" mode
- Decrease blood pressure & heart rate
- Reduce & lower stress & cortisol levels
- Make space to respond instead of react
  - **inhale -** love
  - **pause - in between** feel the love
  - **exhale -** what no longer serves you
  - **pause - in between** feel the release
  - **repeat -** 3 minutes in gratitude a few times a day or more for joy.

Expert 3
Dr. Pat Buchanan
Back Pain or Comfort: It's Your Choice

Most back pain results from daily movement choices. Use the following information to make better decisions for more back comfort and less back pain.

1. Your spine has 24 moving bones (vertebrae) separated by discs. Nerves pass between them. Connective tissues control their position. Muscles guide their movement.
2. If you stack your vertebrae like blocks, you use little effort to stay upright. If not, your muscles and other structures have to do more to keep you from falling.
3. Poor alignment causes pain due to muscle fatigue, tissue strain, pressure on nerves, etc. Over time, this leads to chronic pain and reduced function.
4. Doing an activity, like sitting, for long periods creates stiffness, wear and tear, fatigue, and pain.
5. Your sensory system provides useful information to you. Pay attention to its early warnings and adjust your position and movement to find ease and comfort.

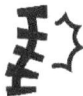

What Will You Choose?

Every day you have choices to make that create habits that either leads to back pain or comfort.

Top 5 back pain habits

- Slouching with your back rounded and tail tucked while sitting or standing
- Positioning your head forward of your torso in sitting or standing
- Standing with your knees locked, which increases pelvic tilt and backpressure
- Sitting for hours at a time
- Ignoring discomfort and pain signals

Top 5 back comfort habits

- Aligning yourself like a stable stack of blocks in sitting and standing
- Centering your head over your torso in sitting and standing
- Unlocking your knees in standing so your pelvis and low back are neutrally aligned
- Breaking from sitting every 30 minutes
- Paying attention and adapting for comfort

To learn more about back comfort habits, go to www.DrPatBuchanan.com/BackComfortHabits.

Expert 4
Deborah Chelette-Wilson
Transforming Trauma Into Triumph

In the aftermath of traumatic experiences, you need safety to express, process, and integrate those experiences. Without a safe, knowledgeable person to help you navigate your experience, you may encounter long-term problems. Symptoms can range from:

1. irritability to rages,
2. sleeplessness to oversleeping,
3. difficulty focusing to focusing on everything and
4. feeling disconnected from yourself and others.

Traumatic stress reactions may happen right away or be delayed. When they are delayed it is difficult to make the connection to the event from long ago to the reactions triggered in the present with no evidence of threat.

1. The younger a person's age the stronger trauma's message can be written outside conscious awareness impacting normal childhood development.
2. Your body is stuck in a low-level state of alarm, easily triggered into reacting as though the experience is happening in the present.

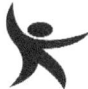

Ways To Turn Trauma Into Triumph

- Find someone who understands the impact of trauma and the need to go at your pace.
- You can't talk your way out of trauma. The experience of trauma impacts your body, mind, emotions and spirituality. You need at times to "feel" your way through.
- Work with someone who can give you an upgrade about your hard-wired attachment and survival systems and what they do after traumatic events.
- Yoga has been found to be a helpful way to release physical tension.
- Learning to self-care is vital to your progress.
- You can learn and practice techniques that will help you self-regulate and take charge of your trauma reactions.
- All of these things can help you triumph over trauma's aftermath.
- Trauma does not have to be a life sentence; but you do need the right guide to light your way.

Deborah Chelette-Wilson, is a Professional Counselor, Belief Detective, Life and Parent Coach
deborah@boundlessfreedoms.com
http://boundlessfreedoms.com

Expert 5
Karen Daniels
Navigate Life With Inner Wisdom

Inner wisdom is a guiding intuition, a knowing that develops throughout your lifetime, perhaps shaped by influential teachers, coaches, relationships, and ideas. Sometimes it has a subtle presence. Allow inner wisdom to sink in. It is natural to be drawn outward. However, with practice, your inner wisdom can be a guiding compass.

1. Take some time to identify mentors, coaches, inspirational people, books, and movies.
2. Determine a few messages or values that each inspirational connection has offered you; things that still stay with you. Write them down. Read them.
3. Practice being still, quiet, and mindful of your body, mind and spirit.
4. Breathe while being aware you are breathing.
5. Create time each week or day to express yourself through writing, moving, doodling, making art, or music.

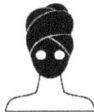

Connect to Inner Wisdom

Connecting inwards can influence your health habits and choices about your life directions.

- Get practiced at noticing when you are being pulled outwards for answers and then stop, find stillness, and turn inward.
- Try selecting an image in your mind to help with self-understanding. For example, if you described your experience of letting go with the image "it's like a melting ice cube" it would be a different way of seeing your situation than "it's like a leaf floating in a wandering stream". Both are moving stories, but with different messages.

Strategies that access imagination can be healing.

- The literary, performing and visual arts, offer many opportunities to tune in to what we love and know.
- Try drumming your rhythm, noticing where your gaze goes in a painting, or choosing a line in a poem that delights you. The discoveries may be surprising. Get more involved in this exciting process. Interested in learning more? Contact me at:
http://www.windsongexpressivearts.com/

Expert 6
Debra Graugnard
Food, Weight & Feminine Power

Subconscious thoughts, beliefs, memories, and feelings have as much impact on your ability to have a body you can love as do your efforts for controlling diet and exercise. A significant contributor to unhealthy subconscious programming is a misperception about the feminine – what it truly means to be a woman.

Here are 5 common beliefs that surface when uncovering such subconscious programming.

1. If I become attractive, I might attract unwanted sexual attention, and that is not safe. I'd better put the weight back on.
2. If I start feeling sexy and spunky, I don't trust myself or who I might become.
3. I feel shame around sexuality and sensuality of the feminine as it is portrayed in the culture.
4. I feel disgust and/or anger about what society expects a woman to be and I don't want any part of it.
5. I feel disconnected from my body and the earth, and I need to eat to reconnect.

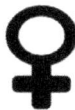

♀

The Truth of the Feminine

Society inundates us with unhealthy pictures of the feminine that do not honor the truth of what a woman is created to be. When you know and honor the true nature of your sacred creation, you will naturally and holistically care for yourself, and your body will respond in a way that is perfect for you uniquely.

Here are some Sacred truths about the Woman. Use these as affirmations when you are feeling doubt, fear, or uncertainty:

- I am a sacred being, with gifts and abilities inherent in my creation that are extremely powerful, beyond the power of this earthly realm.
- I am worthy of love, honor, and respect – no less than that – from anyone, including myself!
- My divine essence is a bridge between the worlds, a bridge to Source.
- I carry the wisdom of earth and spirit. I am a nurturer and protector of life, a knower and connector of the subtle realms, with true power and strength beyond worldly physical strength.
- These are truths of existence. They do not change regardless of what I have done or not done in my life or what I may sometimes believe about myself.

Expert 7
Patty Hedrick RN
Your Roadmap to Active Aging

Aging is inevitable, but you have a choice whether to embrace aging and prepare or bury your head in the sand. It's never too late to begin your journey to a healthy lifestyle.

1. **Mindset and Attitude** - Recent studies prove your mindset determines your age and the elderly can benefit from practicing mindfulness. Focus your mind on the present to practice mindfulness.

2. **Health and Habits** - Set a daily routine for your mind, body, and soul. You have the biggest influence on your health. Take control of your health. Small changes make a big difference, i.e losing only 5 percent of your body weight will greatly improve your overall health.

3. **Planning Ahead** - It is critical to prepare beforehand, and advisable to get professional guidance to prepare a care plan and documents readily accessible for when they are needed.

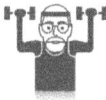

A few recommendations include:

Mindset and Attitude
- Mindfulness exercises including guided imagery, mindful movement, and limiting access to negative news and people.
- Think positively about aging.
- Maintain connections and keep an active social life both on and offline.

Health and Habits
- A daily routine for your mind, body, and soul to keep you fit and healthy.
- Stay curious and never stop learning. Use it or lose it. Challenge your brain.

Planning Ahead - Advanced Care Planning
- Healthcare Documents like insurance information, advance directives, medical release forms, last wishes, etc.
- Financial/Legal Documents like banking information, Power of Attorney, etc.
- Household and Personal Documents like personal identification, passport, contacts, passwords, etc.

To learn more about aging well, go to www.activeaging365.com and get our free checklist and additional support and resources.

Expert 8
Zadra Ibañez
All Essential Oils are Not Created Equal

Many people are turning to essential oils (EOs) to assist with their wellness goals. As more people discover the value of these gifts from nature, companies are cropping up to capitalize on the market. But not all EOs are created equally. Here are some things to look for when you are choosing an essential oil.

1. Essential oils are compounds from plants: stems, roots, leaves, flowers that plants use as natural defenses. These are very useful to people.
2. Essential oils can be used Aromatically, Topically, and in some cases, Internally.
3. Essential oils come in different grades: aromatic, food-grade ("generally recognized as safe" or GRAS,) and therapeutic. You are looking for therapeutic oils to help with health goals and prevention.
4. In order to guarantee that you have the best experience, you need the oils to be complete; meaning, all of the chemical constituents found in the plant are present in the oil.

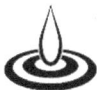

Important things to Know about Oils.

- You need the oil to be pure; free of adulteration or fillers.
- An oil's strength and, therefore, potency can be affected by the climate the plant was grown in.
- The geographic location and also surrounding factors (e.g. is the field next to a freeway?) will impact the results you get from your oil.
- Was the plant harvested at the correct time in its growth cycle?
- Is the oil completely natural, or is it made up of synthetic chemicals?

A few housekeeping items:

- Never put essential oils in plastic containers, i.e. plastic water bottles. The oil will interact with the plastic and you will end up ingesting the plastic molecules. These are the very things you are trying to flush from your body!
- If an oil is "hot," for example oregano or cinnamon oil, you may want to dilute it using a carrier oil or base. Good options are coconut or almond oil, or any milk. Never use mineral oil! Water will spread the oil faster and make it "hotter," because oil and water do not mix, so do not try to flush it with water. Instead, pour milk or oil on a paper towel and pat the area until comfortable.

Expert 9
Joyce Khoury
Understanding the Complicated Medicare Maze

The world of Medicare comes with various rules, enrollment periods, and penalties. Here are some important tools and tips so you can develop a safe way to protect yourself through life's unexpected "*Medicare*" adventures.

1. When you become eligible for Medicare you will need to apply for Part B of Medicare which provides coverage for all medical services and supplies, *but only up to 80% of the cost*. And, if you do not apply for Part B within the required time period you will incur a permanent penalty.

2. You are also required to apply for Medicare Part D, prescription drug coverage or you will be charged with a permanent penalty.

3. If you are employed and turning 65, Part B is optional if your employer offers health insurance. But, be aware! Certain conditions apply.

4. Retiree insurance and *COBRA* are not creditable coverage and you may incur a penalty.

5. There are two types of Medicare coverage: Medicare Supplement Plans and Medicare Advantage Plans.

Important Medicare Facts to Remember

- Medicare has different enrollment periods throughout the year.
- If you do not sign up for Part B and D of Medicare when you become eligible you will incur a permanent penalty which gets larger the longer you delay signing up.
- Retiree insurance and *COBRA* is not creditable coverage.
- *TRICARE* is medical insurance for active-duty military, retirees, and families. If you are a military retiree you must still apply for Part B and pay premiums to keep your *TRICARE* coverage.
- Your contributions to the FICA tax system (Federal Insurance Contributions Act tax) pay for Part A of Medicare as long as you worked and contributed to FICA for a minimum of 10 years or 40 quarters.

Navigating through the Medicare Maze can be daunting and I highly recommend that once you become eligible to receive Medicare benefits you contact a Medicare specialist to help you understand your best options.

The service of a Medicare Specialist is FREE!

Expert 10
Yvonne L Larson
Resilience Mastery

Resilience Mastery is the consistent ability to utilize your whole brain. Without this ability, you work harder, delaying the results you desire.

Understanding Your Resilience Zone:

1. Your Autonomic Nervous System
2. The Function of Your Brain
3. Stress Response: Purpose/Paradox
4. When Default Becomes Dysfunction
5. How & Where Dysfunctions Manifest
6. Mastering Your Resilience

Harness the power of your Resilience Zone and thrive in peak performance flow. In your genius, you fully access clarity, inspiration, focus, and creativity. In this state, you will live a life of success and fulfillment, with efficiency, ease, and grace.

1. Without resilience zone mastery, often multiple patterns are being triggered and perpetuated.
2. Outside support and strategy from a mentor may help to define, distinguish, and design a solution.

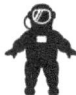

Master Your Resilience/Genius Zone

- Your Autonomic Nervous System is the system regulating your Relaxation Response (R.R.) & Stress Response (S.R.)
- Your S.R. ensures safety & survival.
- When your S.R. activates, your higher cognitive brain functions are diminished.
- The 3 functions of your brain are (1) Regulatory (2) Emotional (3) Cognitive
- Constant stimulation of your S.R. is the paradox of perceiving danger everywhere
- This default state of hyperarousal/ Chronic Stress causes dysfunctional patterns.
- These patterns manifest in 4 areas: Physical, Emotional, Mental, & Spiritual.
- Take the Resilience Mastery Test to Identify your own level of mastery and your next growth edge to catapult your success.
- To get aligned with YOUR GENIUS partner with a Resilience Mastery Strategist!

Yvonne L Larson
Resilience Mastery Strategist
TEST: http://YourResilienceMastery.com
FB: http://ResilienceMasteryGroup.com

Expert 11
Joanne Neweduk
Improving Your Life with Light

Light is an essential nutrient of life. As essential as the air you breathe, the water you drink, and the food you eat. The energy of light (called photons) can be used to improve health and wellness and supports your body's self-healing ability.

1. Sunlight has been used to improve health for thousands of years.
2. Light therapy devices are available for both clinical and home use.
3. Light therapy is known by many names: Photo-biomodulation (PBMT), Polychromatic Light Therapy (PLT), Low-Level Light Therapy (LLLT) and LED therapy to name a few.
4. PBMT is gaining global recognition in numerous health industries as a safe, non-invasive, and non-pharmaceutical therapy with many possible applications.
5. Light triggers the release of nitric oxide in the body which is an important part of your natural healing process and vital to vascular health.

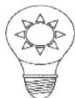

Improving Your Life with Light

Light therapy has many uses and applications. Scientific literature demonstrates that PBMT has the ability to:

- Decrease inflammation in the body, Inflammation is responsible for many of today's ailments,
- Relieve local pain
- Promote relaxation
- Increase circulation - reduce edema
- Improve wound healing.

When finding a practitioner or choosing a light therapy machine for your own use:

- Ensure the practitioner or distributor is knowledgeable and qualified.
- Choose a machine that pulses the light as studies show this has greater benefit.
- Find a well-established manufacturer.

It is conceivable that in the future, every home will have a light therapy machine just as we have a T.V. and computer.

To learn more about light therapy and other stress-reducing modalities visit www.FabulousHealth.ca

Expert 12
Denise Schickel, Ph.D
Your Body

"The body never lies."
~Martha Graham

It is through your body that you experience your life. The healthier your body the better you will feel.

1. Your body has its own needs and desires. Listen to it.
2. You have a body entrusted to you in this life; it is up to you what you do with it.
3. Everyone ages. You cannot avoid it. You can preserve your body with care.
4. Accept your body as it is.
5. Experience your body from the inside out, not from the outside image in.
6. Your body is home base. Without your, body you are nowhere.

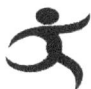

Your Body

"Let the inner god that is in each one of us speak. The temple is your body, and the priest is your heart: it is from here that every awareness must begin."

~Alejandro Jodorowsky

- Your body is your primary vehicle.
- All living organisms grow, bloom, mature, and age. Your body is a living organism.
- Your body transmutes - food into energy, experiences into feelings and thoughts.
- Have fun with your body – through adornment, fashion, movement, and self-expression.
- Your body is an opportunity to express yourself through art.
- Your body connects your spirit to the material world.
- What other people think about your body is not your concern.
- Your body is your own personal action figure.
- What you do with your body is your business.

Expert 13
Patricia Tanner, CR
Health Benefits of Essential Oils
Clarity – Focus – Memory - Calm

All Business Entrepreneurs struggle with the issues listed in this chapter. There is help and it is SO EASY!!!

1. New USB Essential Oil Diffusers plug into your laptop or your main pc and you can carry them with you as well with a USB charger.
2. They are a Wonderful invention to use while you are very busy growing and managing your business.
3. One essential oil from Young Living (YL), "Clarity", can be used to keep your thoughts from going off into a southern detour.
4. YL "Peace and Calming" is for that time when you're working on something stressful or new, staying the course, and feeling accomplished when meeting a goal.
5. YL "Rosemary" is used for memory; a favorite when working on pulling several reports and pieces of information together; to not forget important critical pieces of a report.
6. YL "Brain Power" is another of the memory essential oils to assist in clarity.

Other uses for your USB diffuser:

- Children doing homework
- Relaxation
- Health
    - Asthma
    - Chest colds
    - Trauma
    - Air purification in place of artificial air spray products.

And this is only just a shortlist of all the health benefits of essential oils.

Learn more – follow me on:

Young Living Essential Oils
65 Going On 45
It's not about your age – It's about your health

http://MYYL.com/Tannerhealth

Expert 14
Denise Thomson
How Does Stress Increase Disease?

Stress is defined as an illness that affects a person, animal, or plant. (Webster's Dictionary) 75 – 90% of all doctor's office visits are for stress-related ailments and complaints such as headaches, high Blood Pressure, heart problems, diabetes, skin conditions, asthma, arthritis, depression, and anxiety. OSHA claims that stress in the USA alone costs more than $300 billion annually.

1. Exercise daily to reduce stress.
2. Eat healthy
3. Hydrate properly
4. Live a life in harmony and balance
5. Play relaxing music or spend time with a close friend for help in relieving your stress.
6. Don't dwell on things you cannot change.
7. Yesterday is History, tomorrow is a Mystery, today is a gift - that's why it's called the Present. Live in the present, do, give, and be your best daily!

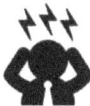

Tips to avoid or reduce stress-related disease

- Choose between stress-causing disease or a happy and relaxed life increasing health.
- You are in control. Don't allow others to take your control away from you.
- Love yourself. You cannot love yourself and create stress at the same time. Stress is a reflection of how you perceive things or yourself.
- Take care of yourself first; schedule time daily, so you are energized and living in harmony.
- Send stress on its way and fend off disease with harmony, authenticity, being true to yourself.

Expert 15
Ronni Zorn
VITAL, VIBRANT & VIVACIOUS
WITH VEGGIES

Eating vibrant, colorful fresh vegetables can help you live a longer, healthier more fulfilling life. You can have a healthier heart and arteries, lower blood sugar, cholesterol, and blood pressure, have more energy, and a BETTER SEX LIFE.

1. Eat a large salad daily & more plant-based whole food meals.
2. But where will I get my protein?
3. Without milk I won't get enough calcium.

The benefits of eating a whole-food plant-based (WFPB) lifestyle is well documented, revealing:
-Vegetables are loaded with vitamins, minerals, antioxidants, & healthy fiber.
-Eating raw dark green leafy vegetables releases nitric oxide, which when combined with our saliva, heals the lining of blood vessels, improving circulation.
-Eating more vegetables, less animal protein and fat, and less refined and processed foods:
- helps you lose weight & improves energy
- reduces blood sugar
- improves brain function
- reduces the risk and can even reverse cardiovascular disease, and erectile dysfunction.

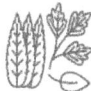

Answers to your questions about a Whole Food Plant-Based Diet.

In the Blue Zones, areas of the world where people live the longest, people follow a whole foods plant-based lifestyle and have the oldest population without disease in the world.

- Drs. Barnard, Essylstyn, Ornish, and Fuhrman advocate eating a large salad with the colors of the rainbow daily.

Where will I get my protein?

- Pound per pound dark green leafy vegetables and many other veggies contain more absorbable and digestible protein per pound than animal protein.
- Eating a pound of a plant-based meal uses significantly less water and energy to produce than a 1/2lb of hamburger.
- Eating more plant-based meals saves animal's lives while reducing your carbon footprint.

The only way I can get calcium is by eating cheese and yogurt, and drinking milk.

- Foods like broccoli, kale, kidney beans almonds, sesame and chia seeds, collard greens, and oranges are rich in calcium easily absorbed and utilized by the body.
- We consume more dairy in the US than any other country on the planet, yet we continue to have the highest incidence of osteoporosis.

You've finished. Before you go...

Tweet/share that you finished this book.

Please star rate this book.

Reviews are solid gold to writers. Please take a few minutes to give us some itty bitty feedback.

ABOUT THE AUTHORS

Donna Bach and Gary Groesbeck are an experienced team whose mission is to assist clients in discovering the optimal states of "Flow or Peak Experiences". Training your own brainwaves leaves no guesswork for getting into the desired frequencies. Virtual training online is also available on their website- www.neuroalchemyflow.com.

Sharon Barnard is a Holy Yoga instructor certified in yoga nidra (yogic sleep), trauma sensitive, and yin yoga. She lives in Orange County, California and hosts classes, events, workshops, and retreats. For a FREE PICTURE OFFICE YOGA PDF request it at: sharonbarnard@holyyoga.net or www.inhaleloveyoga.com

Pat Buchanan, Ph.D. is a movement improvement expert, speaker, and author who helps people stop struggling with physical pain and start living healthier, happier, and more productive lives. Dr. Pat has helped thousands of people, from high-level athletes to children with neurological conditions, improve their movement during her 40+ years working in university, clinic, research, and private settings.

Deborah Chelette-Wilson is a Texas Licensed Professional Counselor and Life and Parenting Coach.

Karen Daniels; With an enthusiasm for imaginative expression, Karen Daniels inspires wellness through the arts.

Debra Graugnard is a best-selling Author, Speaker, and a Master Healer and teacher in the Shaddhiliyya Sufi Order. Through her transformational programs and retreats, Debra guides people to experience the joy of their Divine Essence and live true to their most authentic Sacred Selves.

Patty Hedrick RN, is a Healthcare Consultant with over 30 years of experience navigating through the healthcare system and helping others achieve their highest level of independence by offering guidance, support, and resources. She enjoys working as a Nurse Entrepreneur, speaking, traveling, and spending time with family and friends.

Zadra Rose Ibañez has used essential oils and home-based remedies all her life and has been teaching best essential oil practices for over sevenyears. Her focus is the science behind why and how oils work for people.

Joyce Khoury Born in New Bedford, Massachusetts, currently lives in Santa Monica, California holds a license in Life & Health Insurance, and is also a licensed Real Estate Broker. Joyce's various job experiences have helped her gain a tremendous understanding of how to help people, and today she finds her career as a Medicare Insurance Specialist one of the most satisfying endeavors of her life.

Yvonne L Larson is an International Podcast Host, Resilience Strategist, Master Healer, and the inventor of the Genius Activation Sequence™. She teaches Entrepreneurs struggling from anxiety, fear, and overwhelm how to get connected, stay focused, and sustain their energy so they Thrive In Their Genius and experience success AND fulfillment in all aspects of their personal and professional life.

Joanne Neweduk was born to lead, nurture, and promote vibrancy. A registered nurse, multi-modality wellness innovator, author, coach, and podcaster; she is also the CEO of FabulousHealth and Fabulous at 50.

Denise Schickel has worked for over 30 years as a massage therapist. This experience, along with her Ph.D. in Organizational Psychology, has informed her development of Self-Care Strategies.

Patricia Tanner is a Certified Reflexologist, CNHP Nutritional Consultant, and Aroma Therapy practitioner. Having been in Alternative Health for over 25 years she has always enjoyed the satisfaction of being able to help people feel better.

Denise Thomson is a Certified Health and Wellness Coach, nurse, fitness trainer, educator, speaker, and Bestselling author who loves guiding others to their optimal health. She leads by example, as she has been there, done that, and is maintaining her health by being her best.

Ronni Zorn is a chiropractor with certifications in digestive enzymes, sports injury, plant based-nutrition, and extensive training in nutrition and health and wellness coaching. She loves helping people map out a doable plan to achieve their health and wellness goals.

If you enjoyed this Itty Bitty® Book you might also like…

- **Your Amazing Itty Bitty® Business Experts Compilation Book** – Various Authors

- **Your Amazing Itty Bitty® Holistic Experts Compilation Book** – Various Authors

- **Your Amazing Itty Bitty® Book of Words** – Various Authors

And many other Itty Bitty® Books available on line at www.ittybittypublisihing.com.